# EXERSEXOLOGY

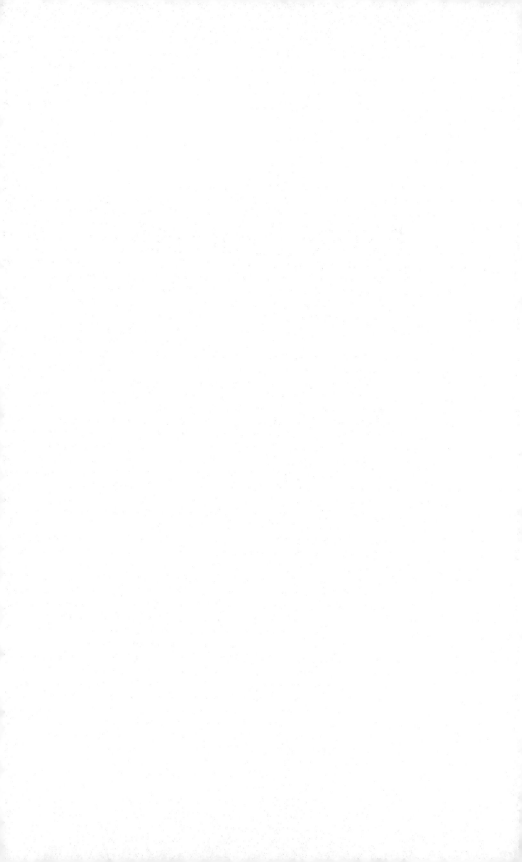

# EXERSEXOLOGY

## The study of calorie burn during sex

# Monique Hollowell

iUniverse, Inc.
Bloomington

# Exersexology
## The study of calorie burn during sex

*Disclaimer:* The information in this book is meant to supplement, not replace proper exercise training. All forms of exercise pose some inherent risk. The editors and publishers advise readers to take full responsibility for their safety and know their limits. The exercises in this book are not intended to substitute for any exercise routine that may have been prescribed by your doctor. As with all exercise programs you should get your doctors approval before beginning. Mention of specific companies, organizations, or authorities in this book does not imply endorsement by the publisher, nor does mention of specific companies, organizations, or authorities imply that they endorse this book. Internet addresses and telephone numbers given in this book were accurate at the time it went to press.

iUniverse books may be ordered through booksellers or by contacting:

iUniverse
1663 Liberty Drive
Bloomington, IN 47403
www.iuniverse.com
1-800-Authors (1-800-288-4677)

Because of the dynamic nature of the Internet, any web addresses or links contained in this book may have changed since publication and may no longer be valid. The views expressed in this work are solely those of the author and do not necessarily reflect the views of the publisher, and the publisher hereby disclaims any responsibility for them.

Any people depicted in stock imagery provided by Thinkstock are models, and such images are being used for illustrative purposes only.
Certain stock imagery © Thinkstock.

ISBN: 978-1-4759-6354-0 (sc)
ISBN: 978-1-4759-6355-7 (ebk)

Printed in the United States of America

iUniverse rev. date: 12/04/2012

# Introduction _____

As a fitness expert I am always asked the question: 'What are the best ways to burn calories?' I often give the calorie burning advice of walking, running, jump roping, swimming, etc. But one key calorie burning exercise that we tend to forget is sex! Sex is an important part of my life and I truly feel it should be an integral part of yours. Therefore, as your fitness expert, I want to show you how sex can improve your overall fitness!

So how many calories do we actually burn during sex? In a recent article titled, '8 surprising health benefits of sex,' by Women's Day Magazine, Desmond Ebanks, MD founder and medical director of Alternity Healthcare in West Hartford, Connecticut quoted, "sex burns between 75-150 calories per half-hour," which is comparable to other types of exercise activities such as walking (153 calories per half-hour) or dancing (129 calories per half-hour). So guess what? More sex, burns more calories!

Dr. Ebanks also expressed many other health benefits of sex such as:

- Sex is exercise that raises heart rate and blood flow. In a study published in the Journal of Epedemiology and Community Health, researchers found that having sex twice per week reduced the risk of fatal heart attack by half
- Sexual arousal and orgasm releases the hormone testosterone, which, among other things, is necessary to build and maintain bone and lean muscle tissue

- People having frequent sex often report that they handle stress better. Many indicate that they sleep more deeply and restfully after satisfying love making
- Individuals who have sex once or twice per week show 30 percent higher levels of an antibody called Immunoglobin A, which is known to boost the immune system (study by researchers at Wilkes University in Pennsylvania)

So not only is sex fun and something that we enjoy, but sex also brings a great addition to your overall health and fitness.

# The Founding Concept _____

As funny as this may seem, my concept of Exersexology™ first came about through a fun, unofficial calorie burning case study, in which I had a select amount of fitness professionals wear calorimeters/heart rate monitors (devices which can track heart rate and calorie burn during physical activities, the device can be worn around the arm, wrist or chest) to see accurate calories burned for different lifestyles and activities. Within 2 weeks of the case study, some of the fitness professionals wore the devices while having sex? So the curiosity spread like wild fire and before I knew it, I received more off the record data about sex and calories versus calories and lifestyle? This absolutely amazed me for two reasons: first, how hooked individuals became on knowing the exact number of calories burned during sex (which I now call sexisodes) & second: how much more sex the participants were having because of it!

So years past, and I hosted an internet radio show which discussed fitness and sex, and the show was my highest downloaded podcast! At that point I knew it was time to create a new wave of calorie burning sex through Exersexology™.

I want to say thank you to the couples who participated in my calorie burning sex study! The couples utilized heart rate monitors to gather data for each sexisode (sexisode was conducted at least twice with recorded data). All the data was collected and averaged in the final publication of Exersexology™.

Note: The approximate calories burned for each chapter are expressed as kcals, for example, ~162kcals (based upon all positions conducted in the sexisode (i.e chapter)). Everyone's body is completely different and your calorie burn per sexisode may be greater or less than the approximate calorie burn indicated in the sexisode chapter.

For more information and/or to log your results, go to www.exersexology.com. We want to hear from you.

Have fun and enjoy!

Bring your *'A' Game*, with this fantastic mix of alpha female and male dominant positions. *'A' Game* will ignite your competitive nature by *giving* ultimate pleasure and *receiving* maximal satisfaction.

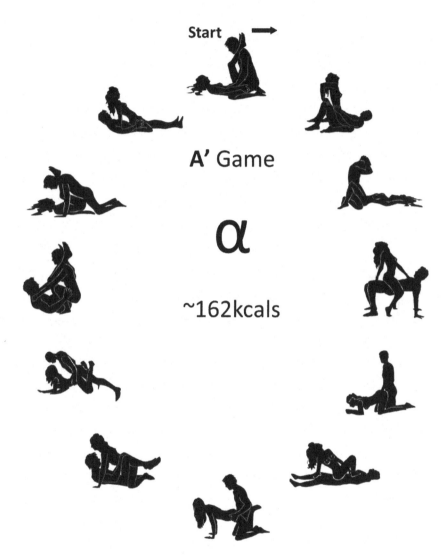

Welcome to your hardcore sex obstacle course of tricky positions. *Bootcamp* is full of angles, oppositions, fun and laughter! This is your ultimate workout full of sweat, sound and humpin' around!

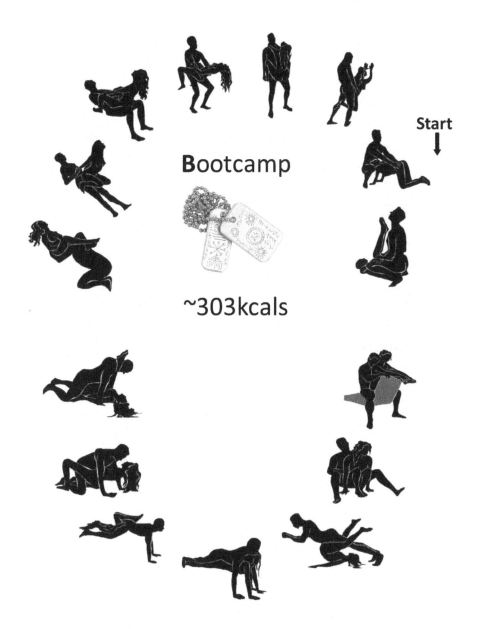

Bootcamp

~303kcals

Start

No time to lie down, let's test your stamina! *Cross walk* consists of standup positions by one or both partners. Get ready for a phenomenal leg and abdominal workout during an all standing sexisode!

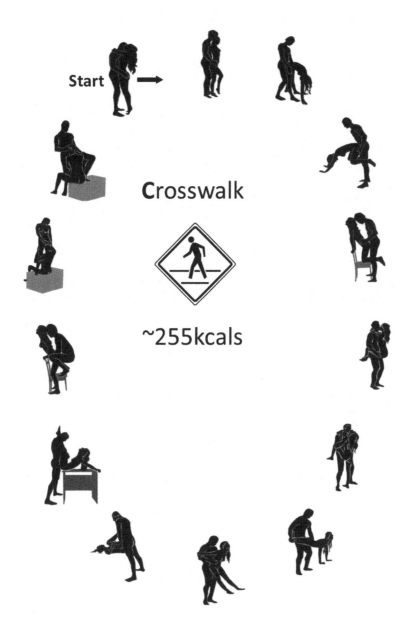

Start

Crosswalk

~255kcals

Admire the mirror image of your partner by performing the same positions on each other. Explore your mutual power to bend, stretch and thrust the body. *Ditto* will answer your most infamous question:

'I wonder what *'it'* feels like, to be in *'that'* position?'

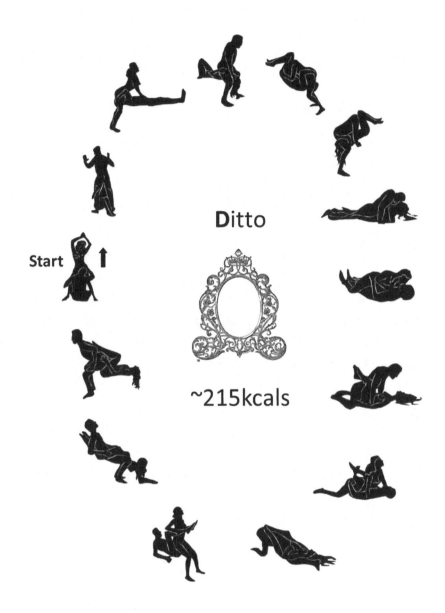

Start

Ditto

~215kcals

Like the slow turn of our world, so is the *Earth* sexisode. The male and female genitalia should stay connected as your bodies gradually move from one position to another. This amazing sexual sequence will have you turning and rotating the entire time.

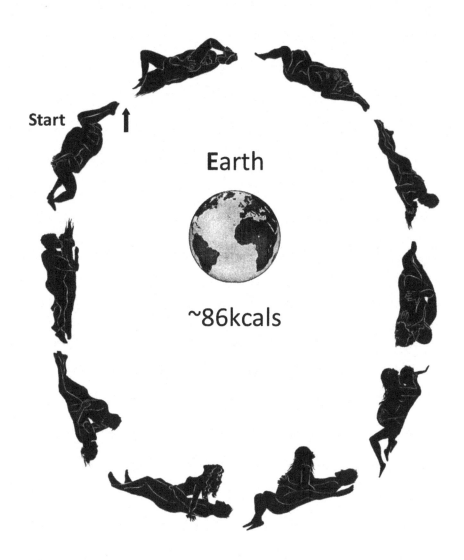

**Start**

Earth

~86kcals

I know you're *Famish*ed, so it's time to eat!

Tap into the pleasures of the mouth and enjoy the eroticism of your oral zone.

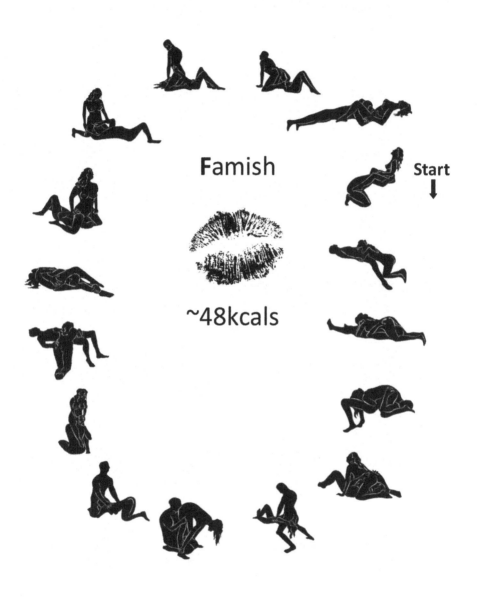

Famish

~48kcals

Start

Get sexified right side up and upside down by defying the earth's gravitational pull. Demonstrate your strength and explore the power of pleasing each other from all angles.

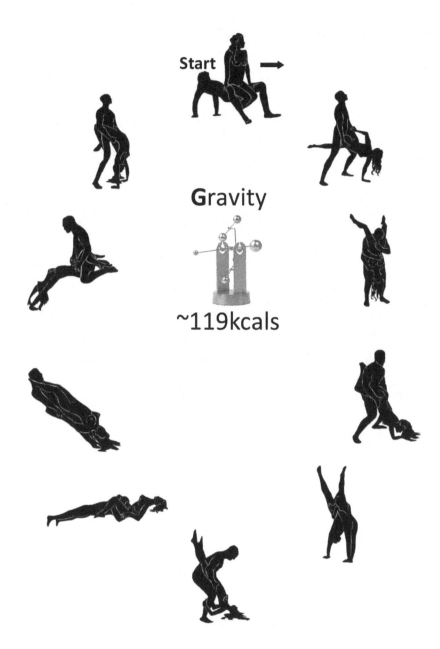

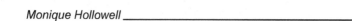

Ladies, how good can you ride? Hop on the saddle and get the ultimate hip, thigh and butt work out. Utilize a fun strap to wrap around the hips and/or the shoulders for the ultimate grip and control, because you don't want to fall off!

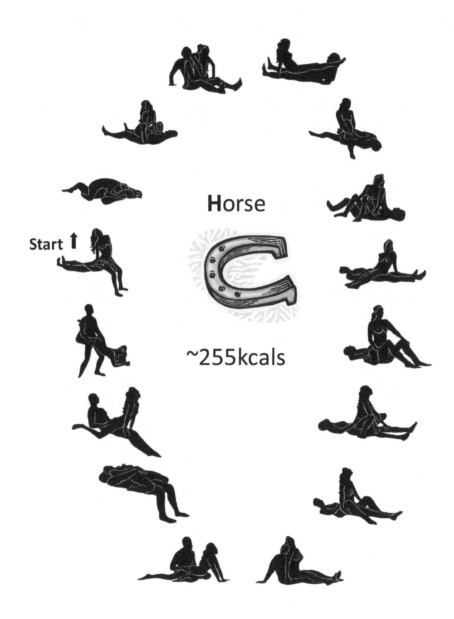

Horse

~255kcals

Start

Get ready for the long haul with 21 exotic positions. Give yourselves at least 90 minutes to ignite your flames with infinite positions to orgasm and calories to burn.

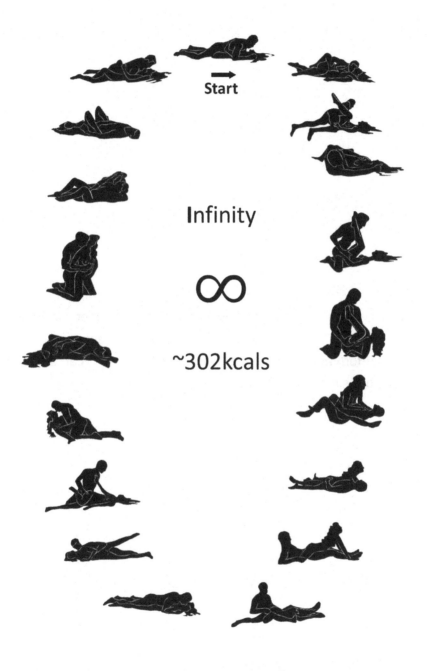

Start

Infinity

∞

~302kcals

Joule is defined as 'the unit of *work* or *energy* in the metric system.' The energy is your body, the work is the sex and the metric system is your performance! Challenge yourselves to see who can burn the most calories with these 10 invigorating positions!

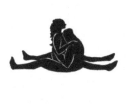

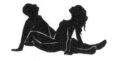

Joule

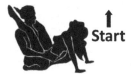

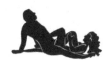

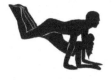

J

↑
Start

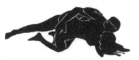

'dʒaʊl'

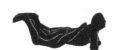

~180kcals

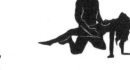

Nothing compares to lusty tangles between each other. Focus on your bodies becoming fully intertwined. It's such a pleasure when every inch of you are twisted up in a knot.

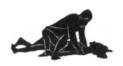

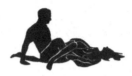

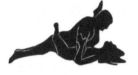

**K**notty

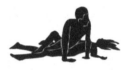

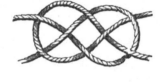

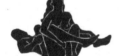

~57kcals

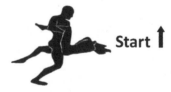

Start ⬆

Overflow and indulge yourself in these 8 positions. Heat up your body to its highest point of passion. Lava will take you through peaks and valleys until you reach your climax, sexplode and let loose your Lava!

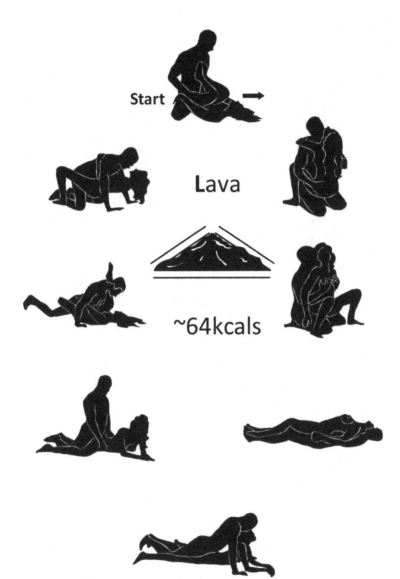

Start

Lava

~64kcals

Mélange is a fun medley of 6 sexual pieces that will give you a calorie burning, puzzle surprise.

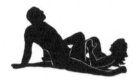

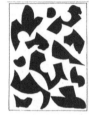

# Mélange

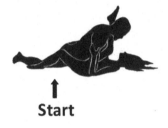

**Start**

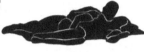

~49kcals

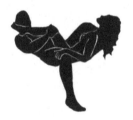

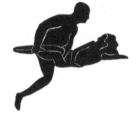

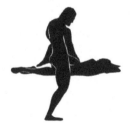

Will you be Naughty or Nice? Let's go with Naughty! Challenge yourselves to balance the pleasure and intensities of these 7 positions. Enjoy the quality of positions versus the quantity of orgasms.

(A Blind fold and tie may come in handy!)

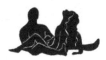

# Naughty or Nice

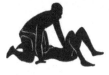

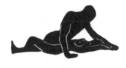

**Start**

~78kcals

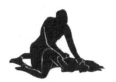

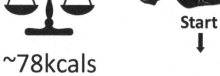

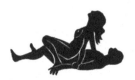

Let's bring out the acrobat in you! *Oscillate* will have your body moving in breath taking directions. You will demonstrate phenomenal upper body and hip strength to achieve your ultimate pleasure.

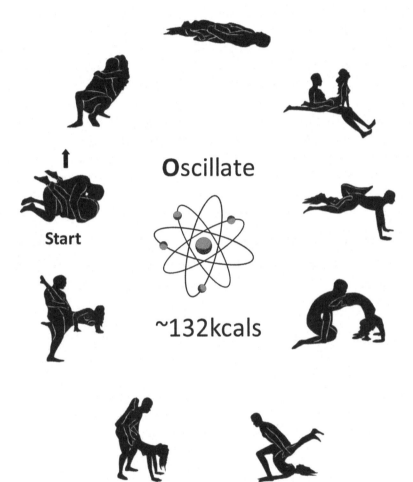

**O**scillate

~132kcals

Start

Allow your body to move in a series of soft angled positions! These 10 dynamic motions come in an array of G-spot pleasures and deep penetration.

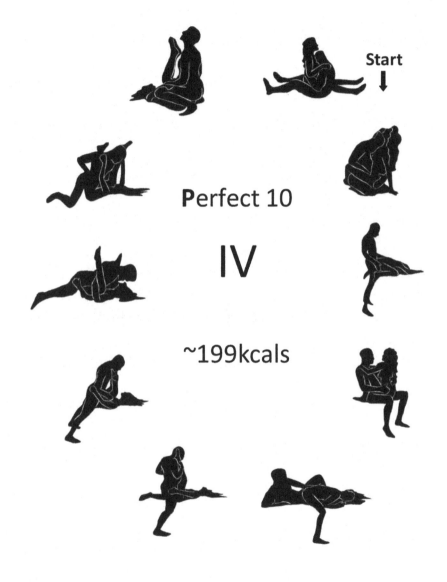

Start

Perfect 10

IV

~199kcals

There is nothing like the beauty of 5 flowing positions which create the ultimate harmony. Make beautiful music together by enjoying the flow and sequence of the *Quintet*. This could be one of your favorites!

**Start**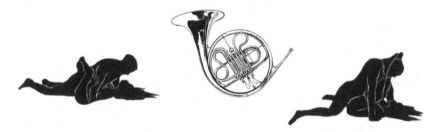

## Quintet

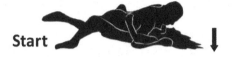

~128kcals

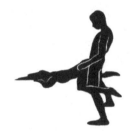
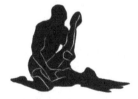

*Rubber band'* will test your flexibility and balance. Both partners will stretch and be stretched in 12 amazing positions. This sexisode will loosen and relax those tight muscles of the legs, hips, back and neck. It's such a pleasure to be stretched, and have an orgasm too!

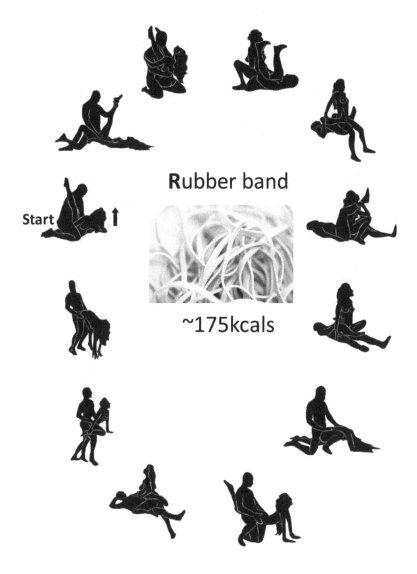

**R**ubber band

~175kcals

Start ↑

Need a quickie? If so, here it is! This sexisode is lower on the calorie burn but great for the 10-15 minute sex ride! The straight shooter is composed of traditional positions to burn some quick energy and satisfy your sexual desires.

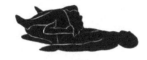

# **S**traight Shooter

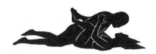

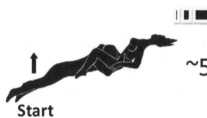

**Start**

~54kcals

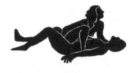

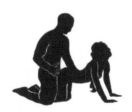

Tic Tac Toe, 3 orgasms in a row! This sexisode is designed to climax every 2 positions with a 7$^{th}$ position for deep penetration (possibly creating a 4$^{th}$ orgasm)! Each position will ignite your ultimate release. Can you handle all 3?

What a fun game to play!

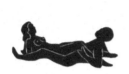

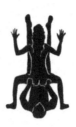

# Tic Tac Toe

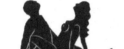

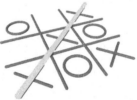

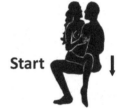

Start ↓

~131kcals

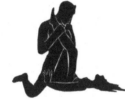

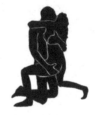

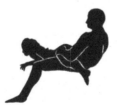

Spread them wide, spread them long and spread them out! Open those limbs and test your flexibility. The Umbrella will unleash pleasure in widespread positions. Allow your partner to take control and spread you beyond your limits.

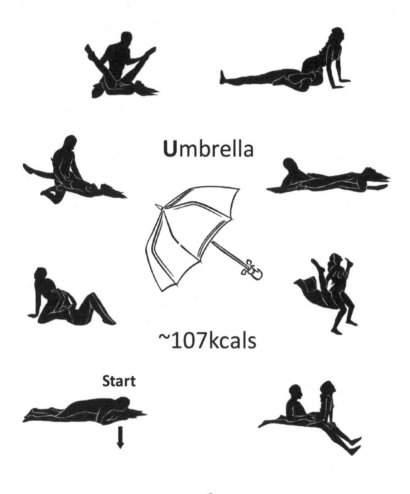

**U**mbrella

~107kcals

Start

Engage yourself in the electrifying intensity of *Voltage*. The short held positions will create quick deep thrust and potent orgasms. Brace yourself for the unique power you'll find behind these 11 positions!

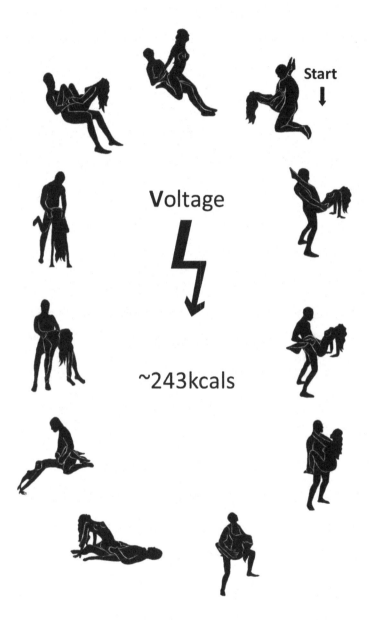

**Start**

Voltage

~243kcals

A poem for you: *'I wish upon a star that you've experienced the best sex so far, but that you're still willing to explore, what the wishbone has in store.'* Ever wished for a sexual episode of bliss and relaxation? **I dare you to try this sexisode in locations other than the bedroom**!

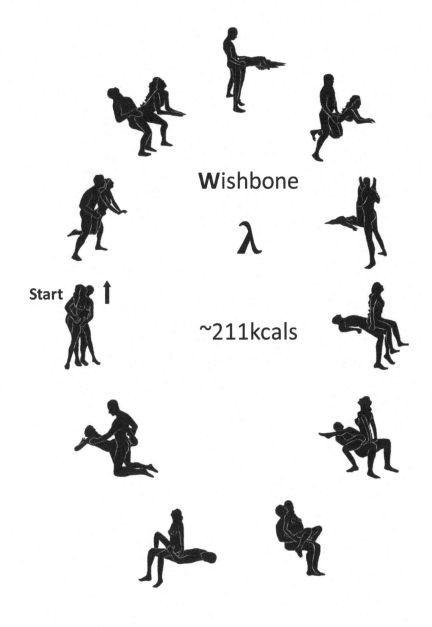

Wishbone

λ

~211kcals

Start ↑

Get x-rated and feel like the star of your own triple x movie. The 11 positions are frequently seen on the erotic circuit. Embrace your own stardom with these positions to win an x-rated award of your own.

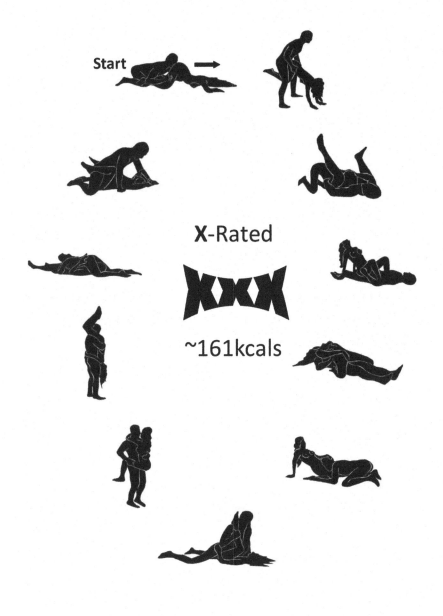

Stay eye to eye to view the pleasures of your partner. Yin n Yang focuses on the front facing positions while alternating of who is on top and who is on bottom.

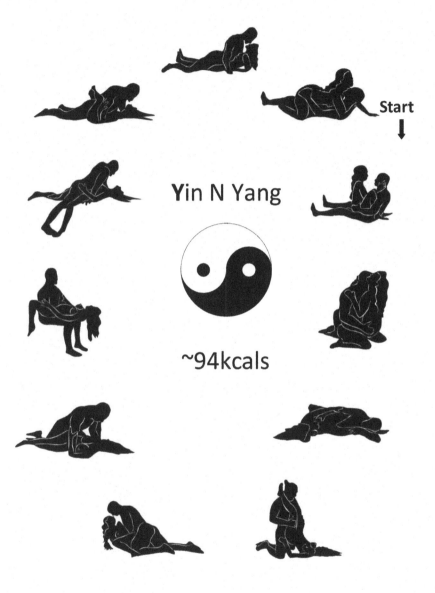

Yin N Yang

Start

~94kcals

# Zodiac

Each zodiac sign has its dominant position in which they give and receive the best! Explore the Zodiac circle and find which position drives your partner to ecstasy. Challenge yourself with all 12 positions of the zodiac circle to decide which sign is your ultimate match. See what the astrology experts have said about you!

## Air Signs (Gemini, Libra and Aquarius): *Fickle lovers*

A healthy dose of fantasy goes along way with these heady types, positions which invite the use of imagination are the best.

Favorite positions: Reverse cowgirl or the 'sit down' position (both require one person to be on top of the other) offers unique stimulation for both partners and invite a little adventure without intense eye to eye contact

## Earth Signs: (Taurus, Virgo and Capricorn): *Sensual lovers*

Tend to enjoy athletic sex and anything that keeps them fully engaged.

Favorite positions: Try having sex standing up. Whether one partner is up and against the wall or inverted with the straddling partner bent over backwards

**Water Signs (Scorpio, Cancer and Pisces):** *Deep sexual intensity lovers*

Each has a desire for emotional connection via sexual pleasure.

Favorite positions: CAT (Coital Alignment Technique) main focus is maximum stimulation for both partners. These positions enhance the likeliness of simultaneous orgasms. Missionary position (putting maximal weight into the pelvis) and 'Starfish' (both partners lay back, heads in opposite directions, legs in scissor position)

**Fire Signs: (Aries, Leo, and Sagittarius):** *Animalist lovers*

Fire signs love a sense of adventure and actual conquest; perhaps even aggression.

Favorite positions: Doggie style and 'women on top.' Any position which puts the fire sign in a power position (dominate or be dominated) because they like to be on display

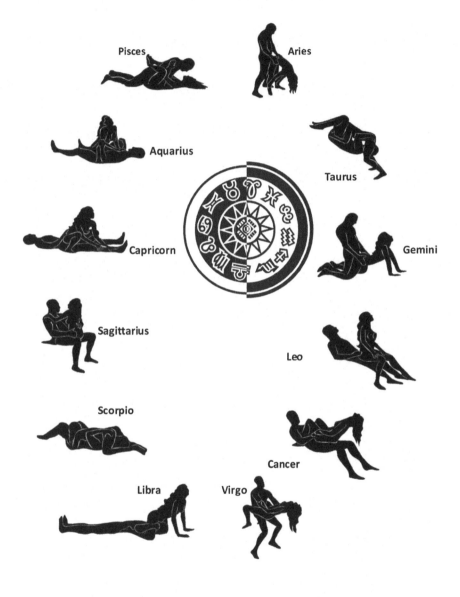

# About the Author

Monique Hollowell has more than 13 years fitness industry experience. She is the author of *Bellie Fit Basics*, a radio show host, national presenter and CEO of Lafemme Mobile Gym. Monique has been featured in multiple radio shows, news segments and national publications such as Ebony and Happen Magazine.